BROKEN

A Journey of Depression and Disbelief

BROKEN

A Journey of Depression and Disbelief

BY

DOUGLAS R. TULL JR

TATE PUBLISHING
AND ENTERPRISES, LLC

Published by Tate Publishing & Enterprises, LLC
127 E. Trade Center Terrace | Mustang, Oklahoma 73064 USA
1.888.361.9473 | www.tatepublishing.com

Tate Publishing is committed to excellence in the publishing industry. The company reflects the philosophy established by the founders, based on Psalm 68:11,
"The Lord gave the word and great was the company of those who published it."

Published in the United States of America

ISBN: 978-1-68028-548-2
1. Religion / Christian Life / Inspirational
2. Medical / Oncology
14.11.11

ENDORSEMENTS AND REVIEWS

By Paula on April 3, 2014

Rated 5 Stars
This was a great book that really brought attention to how someone goes through getting devastating news and bringing God into their life to help get through. It definitely kept my attention!
4.0 out of 5 stars **Broken** January 9, 2014

By WillyP

I enjoyed reading this book. I think anyone who is facing a spiritual battle could benefit from reading this. He shares with the reader his journey from being on top of the world, then finding out he has a terrible illness, and then falling into the deep pit of depression. His struggle with these difficult circumstances ultimately led him to a new outlook on life. This book is his story of finding a true relationship with Christ in the midst of a storm.

4.0 out of 5 stars **so very real for us all...** January 6, 2014

By Judy

Very good short read with the ups and downs of his life. Does he see the real picture? Only God could answer.

ACKNOWLEDGEMENTS &

DEDICATION

I would like to dedicate this book to my amazing wife Tori. Through thick and thin she has stood by me and helped me through the darkest of times. She has always offered me encouragement and support no matter how foolish or ambitious my ideas were. No matter where I am in life I can be sure that she is always standing by my side. I am never alone and for that I am forever grateful. God knew exactly what he was doing when he led us together. He understood my needs and provided me the perfect partner who completes me, controls me, supports me, encourages me, and guides me through all things.

I would also like to say thank you to my two precious sons. Douglas and James you are one of the main reasons I do everything I do. My family is my everything and I am eternally grateful to have the most well behaved and loving sons. They fill my life with joy and happiness. Our home is filled with laughter and love every day. Daddy loves you both.

Lastly I want to say thank you to my family. My mom and dad made me the man I am today and I will be forever thankful. Thank you Kenny and Lori for all that you have given to help me and my family. And thank you to all of my church family, you guys carried me often when I was down.

BROKEN

BROKEN

ACKNOWLEDGEMENTS & DEDICATION

INTRODUCTION

CHAPTER 1

The Start of the Downward Spiral

CHAPTER 2

Battling Leukemia and More

CHAPTER 3

U-Turn

CHAPTER 4

Escape & Visitation

CHAPTER 5

The Encouragers

CHAPTER 6

Cruise Control

CHAPTER 7

Struggling to be disciplined

Chapter 8

The Awakening

Chapter 9

I Will Rise

Broken

A Caregiver's View

INTRODUCTION

As I sit down to write this I find myself in a very unique place. It has been so very difficult over the past few years and I wanted to be able to share my story in hope that I might be able to touch someone else and help them to understand the pain and sorrow that has engrossed them. If you are looking for a book with medical information about how to diagnose or treat some of the illnesses I will discuss then you have come to the wrong place. This is about a journey. About living one day at a time and never giving up. There were times when I felt like giving up all hope; I had to force myself to live. Going to church was a chore and praying was difficult. This book will talk about my ups and downs, the good times and bad, the joys and the sorrows.

I will talk about how to recognize some signs of depression, not clinical terms but the way I felt, the things I did, and how it affected those around me. I will give you scripture references that helped me to stay focused and close to God. Jesus loves me I do believe that and I have felt his presence many times. I will talk about how I was able to recognize him through the darkness and how my family and friends encouraged me and allowed me to live when I wanted to die. I will discuss my leukemia and how it has affected me and my life again nothing technical, but my journey, my emotional rollercoaster, and the triumphs and failures.

You may think that this book is going to be filled with doom and gloom, but I assure you that is not the case. I have had too many good times to stay focused only on the bad things. It has been this ability to control my focus and concentration that keeps me sane. Without the valleys there would be no mountains, and we could not appreciate the magnificence of God's grace if not for the low points from which he rescued us. I hope that my story can bless you and help you to travel through the fiery trials that may arise. You need to know that there is light at the end of the tunnel even though you may not be able to see it right now... it is there. You may feel alone but you're not, and when you think no one cares remember that you are loved beyond unbelievable measure. There is a time for everything just as it states in

Ecclesiastes 3: 1-8 *For everything there is a season, and a time for every matter under heaven: a time to be born, and a time to die; a time to plant, and a time to pluck up what is planted; a time to kill, and a time to heal; a time to break down, and a time to build up; a time to weep, and a time to laugh; a time to mourn, and a time to dance; a time to cast away stones, and a time to gather stones together; a time to* *embrace, and a time to refrain from embracing; a time to seek, and a time to lose; a time to keep, and a time to cast away; a time to tear, and a time to sew; a time to keep silence, and a time to speak; a time to love, and a time to hate; a time for war, and a time for peace.*

You may feel like you are never going to get out of the fog, but believe me that there will be a brighter tomorrow. The sun will rise in the morning. Everything comes and everything goes, for us we have to endure and grow through the process. This endurance will allow us to grow closer to the Lord and develop character that will help us to face the future and find joy and harmony when it appears there is none.

There is never a great time to be sick. There is never joy in finding out you have a disease. And life can appear cold and black, but there is warmth, and love, and happiness to be found in even the most terrifying of situations. When you wake up you have to recognize what is important to you and know that you have a choice as to how you will approach your day. You can choose sorrow and depression, or you can choose hope and joy. Please understand I am not saying that depression is a choice, but I am saying your conscious efforts can help you to rise above the somber weight of depression.

I had many days in which I just wanted to lay there and do absolutely nothing but sulk and pity myself. And to be quite honest many times I did. I chose not to rise above on many occasions. I failed to get up when I fell down. Too often I found myself lost and out of control. Hopefully this book can help you to gain control, to increase your faith, and to overcome the darkness in your life.

CHAPTER 1

The Start of the Downward Spiral

My crazy spiraling journey started a couple of years ago. It was June of 2008 and it was a Thursday. Just like everyone else it was getting close to TGIF. I was happy I had made it to the end of the week and I was looking forward to the weekend. I had been plugging along through the day and had gotten through lunch and it started. I begin to feel a little yucky. I started feeling kind of warm and then my head begin to hurt and my neck started to get stiff. Within just a few hours I was feeling really dizzy and lightheaded. Somehow I ended up extremely ill and was in no condition to drive home, so I called my wife and told her that she was going to have to come and get me and drive me home. I was severely sick and I knew it. Whatever it was it came on fast and furiously. She called the doctor and they agreed to see me after work so she drove to my office and picked me up at four o'clock, we left my car there and she picked it up later.

By the time she got there I was extremely sick. I could barely stand and my head was pounding. I thought for sure I was going to pass out. It was all I could do to walk downstairs to the meet her when she got there. I managed to get to the car and we headed to the doctor's office. When we got there I was so ill she had to help me in to see the doctor. He examined me and sent me straight to the emergency room. So off to the hospital we went. The doctor was concerned I might have meningitis. My fear was really kicking into high gear at this point. The stress level was going through the roof, and I was going downhill fast. At this point and time I was too sick to even be depressed or sad, I was just physically exhausted.

It seemed like the drive to the hospital took forever, I felt every bump in the road and every curve, but we finally got there. We checked in and were taken back to one of the rooms in the emergency area. My fever had climbed to over 104 degrees. They went through the normal motions started an IV, checked my blood pressure, respirations, and ordered some blood work. My blood pressure was up, and my heart rate was racing. Shortly the doctor came in and checked on me and ordered some medication for the headache, requested some x-rays, and told me they were going to do a spinal tap to test for the meningitis. I had been through a couple of spinal taps before and knew what it entailed. I was not looking forward to having a needle stuck into my spine again.

I had had a history of headaches and blackouts. They determined that in the past I had reacted severely to stress and that the blood vessels around my brain would constrict, then my nerves would shut me down so that I wouldn't stroke out. I was getting more and more nervous and the stress level was going up fast. As I lay there in that hospital bed reality begin to set in and I felt like something major was wrong. I just wanted to shut down, make it all go away. How in the world could this be happening? As the stress went up, I physically crashed further and further.

Then the doctor came back with a nurse and I took the necessary position curled up in a ball hugging a pillow, and the procedure was started. He did his best; he made three attempts at the spinal tap, but could not successfully get any flood from the sack around my spinal cord. I was in so much pain and the tears were flowing freely. The doctor gave up and said he wasn't going to torture me anymore. I was thankful for that much. I knew something serious was wrong and the depressed feelings begin to creep in. What was wrong with me? Was I going to die? I was afraid and I didn't know what to do. The doctor apologized and said he would come back as soon as he could with some information.

Thankfully the pain medication was starting to kick in and the throbbing pain in my head started to subside. The stiff neck was still there and I was burning up, but the pounding was gone. The doctor came back shortly and said that the blood work was off and that I was going to be admitted. My white blood count was over forty thousand. They weren't sure what was wrong, but my ticket to hang out was being punched. That was the beginning of seven days of mind numbing insanity.

The next morning an infectious disease specialist came to see me, as did my family doctor. My headaches were ramping up to levels seven and eight and I couldn't stand any light. My temperature was staying over 103 degrees going up to almost 106 degrees. In my mind I just knew I was dying. They begin running a barrage of test including a spinal tap on a tipsy table in the x-ray department, I had cat scans, MRI's, x-rays, and all kinds of other blood work. They tested me for anything and everything, including off the wall things such as diseases you would contract if you had been bitten by a rabbit or goat. I was like, I think I would have remembered that, but whatever you have to do. They begin trying different antibiotics trying to find something that would work but nothing brought any relief.

We were on the cancer floor and a good friend of ours was there with her husband who was in the hospital battling cancer. It was nice because she and my wife, Tori, were able to talk and visit, they could be there for each other through this trial. Whenever her husband was going through a test Tori would go over and be with her and when Tori was struggling she was a strong shoulder for Tori to lean on. It was amazing that God gave them both someone to rely on and talk to for encouragement. It is just as Paul says in **Romans 1: 11-12:** *For I* *long to see you, that I may impart to you some spiritual gift to strengthen you—that is, that we may be mutually encouraged by each other's faith, both yours and mine.* Paul recognized that there was value in being there for one another. Sharing your burdens with others will help keep you from going insane. We are designed to rely on each other sharing our cares and our burdens so that no one succumbs to the weariness and exhaustion that comes with life. Jesus tells us in **Matthew 11: 28-30** *"Come to me, all who labor and are heavy laden, and I will give you rest. Take my yoke upon you, and learn from me, for I am gentle and lowly in heart, and you will find rest for your souls. For my yoke is easy, and my burden is light."*

Sharing allows us to learn from one another and use the experience of one another to make our time in the trial easier. Also when we cast our cares and burdens upon someone stronger they can help to alleviate fears and hurt and allow us to find rest and comfort. Being alone leaves us vulnerable and subject to fear. When our fear is allowed to fester and grow without being held in check than we have no way to control it and what it can do to our minds. And when our mind is being depressed and afraid then our bodies react physically and we face illness and tiredness. We have to be willing to reach out and try to find comfort and help whenever we feel things are too stressful for us to face alone. It is of no use to put up a big strong front. To be honest that is like using super glue to seal cracks in a dam. It simply will not hold for long, eventually the pressure will force its way through and the dam will burst. The void has to be filled with something better and stronger so that it will hold.

I am very thankful that God provided someone to be there for my wife through this time, goodness knows that I was definitely not good company and I was for sure not a good encourager. The one thing I can say is that she never left my side. I am blessed because of that. I know what my marriage means to me today because of the way my wife cared for me then. Unfortunately all of this support did not stop the downward spiral although it did serve to slow it down a little and it gave me footholds to use as I struggled to climb out.

As I lay in that hospital bed through the week so many things went through my mind. Was it a rare and deadly disease? Was I going to die? Who was going to care for my wife and two sons? (I was in the hospital for Father's day). My stress level continued to climb, the headaches continued to worsen, and the fever had yet to break. Then Monday morning rolled around and my family doctor came in to see me. He explained that there was a problem with the blood work. They had found some blast cells in the blood. Basically my white blood count was too high and most of the white blood cells were immature, the immature cells were what they called blast cells. They were calling in an oncologist to see me. I was immediately gripped with fear. I was going to die. I had cancer and I was going to die. I was convinced of that. To say I was depressed would be putting it mildly. I crashed like a two ton truck with no brakes.

Later that morning the oncologist came in and consulted me telling me they were going to do what is known as a bone marrow biopsy. He explained that they would numb the surface of my hip and then drive a spike into my hip bone to get the marrow from the center of the bone. At this point stress and fear went completely through the roof. I did not know what to think or how to react. We prayed and told ourselves this is just precautionary and we aren't going to get upset, but in the back of my mind I was terrified. All I could think was don't let it show. You have to be strong. I felt that if I showed fear then my wife would have no one to depend on and I couldn't let her down. Inside I was slowly degrading and dying, but I was afraid to let it show.

That afternoon the time for the test came. They did the test right there in my room. I rolled over on my right side and gritted my teeth and the oncologist did his thing. I felt the pressure as the spike hit the bone. I heard each tap of the hammer against the spike. Each ping resounding through my head like a thundering clang, I squeezed the pillow and clenched my teeth for all I was worth. The nurse told me how good I was doing, but to tell you the truth I felt like just giving up. I wanted to say no more. Finally it was over and I breathed a sigh of relief and then the doctor tells me that the sample was no good that he would have to do it again to get a better sample. So we had to repeat the entire process. I am not going to lie I wanted to throw that doctor out the window. It hurt too much and I couldn't take it anymore.

Finally it was truly over and they left. I cried and tried to relax but between the pain and the bad thoughts there was no relief. There had been too many problems. I had several reactions in the hospital including one called Red Chief Syndrome. It was the middle of the night and the nurse came in and she looked at me and she went "Oh no!" Those are not words you want to hear coming out of the mouth of your nurse. I was reacting to the antibiotic and it was causing me to swell and turn red and blotchy. They put me on one medication that turned my veins black and was causing them to collapse really badly. There were just so many problems. I just knew this was going to be bad as well. Nothing went well that week and I couldn't see any hope for the future.

Wednesday morning rolled in and things begin to turn around. My fever finally broke and the headache started to lessen. I slowly begin to feel better. Then the oncologist came back in and gave me the news that I was dreading. The test results came back and I had what is called the Philadelphia chromosome. My number 9 and number 22 chromosomes were breaking off and switching places causing my white blood cells to produce in overdrive and release prematurely. I had CML, chronic myelogenous leukemia. I was floored. I had cancer. My mind was racing, my heart was pounding, and I couldn't formulate the most basic of thoughts. What was I going to do? All I could think about was a cousin I had lost years ago to leukemia. I knew I was going to die. I heard very little else that the doctor said that day other than he told me that I had the Cadillac of cancers. I didn't want a Cadillac, I just wanted to go home and wake up from this nightmare. I was so dismayed and distraught nothing was registering.

My wife was so upset she couldn't even say it, she had the doctor write it on a sheet of paper and went out into the hallway and showed it to the wonderful nurse who had been so friendly to us. The nurse treated us like kings. Our friend was there every step re-assuring us that everything would work out. I just sat there in stunned shock. I praise God for that friend because I couldn't reassure my wife, I was unable to be there and be the rock she needed, but God knew that and provided people to be there to care for her.

It didn't take long before the anger set in and I was furious. Why was God doing this to me? I had been faithful, I attended church, I listened to Christian music, and I tried to live according to Biblical standards. What kind of a God would do this to a loyal follower? I didn't want to think about religion, I didn't want to hear about how God would help me, and I didn't want anybody to pray with me or for me. As far as I was concerned God didn't exist and He could take a hike. I didn't want anything to do with God. I was ticked off and I was letting people know it. I was mad enough to chew nails and spit horseshoes, and I would have been spitting ringers at that.

The grieving process had started. I cried and cried. My heart was broken. I wanted to see my boys. I wanted to hug them and kiss them. I just knew that I was a dead man and that I was going to be gone from their lives forever. I couldn't stand the thought of them having to grow up without a father. I begin to beg and plead with my wife to promise that she would marry a good man to raise my sons. I had to figure out how to provide for my family once I was gone, nothing else mattered. I went into planning mode trying to push dealing with the diagnosis off. But I couldn't put it off long. I had to call and notify my family. So I started making the calls. I told my mom and dad, then my sister, and finally I got a hold of my brother at work. I could hear the tears in his voice and I broke. I lost it emotionally. The tears came flooding, the pain swelled, and I wept uncontrollably. We let it all out. Crying and holding each other not talking or thinking, we just were, lost in sorrow and despair.

Finally we begin to calm down and put things into perspective. There were so many questions. What treatments would I have to face? Could I work? Was I going to die? How long did I have? How was I going to tell my boys? Who would care for my family? Would I need special things at home? There were a million questions. The downward spiral was started. I had already lost my grandmother shortly before this and my aunt just found out her cancer was back and was spreading. I lost her shortly thereafter. In total there were eight deaths in my family or inner circle in 2008. People were dropping like flies one was a baby who had been born with health issues, another was my 23 year old cousin who was killed in a car crash, and to me it was logical that my days were numbered. I was going to die it was just a matter of how long until it happened. I was going downhill fast and I couldn't see any hope. My wife looked at me and she asked me straight up "Do you trust Jesus?" I looked at her funny and was like do what. She looked at me and asked me "Do you trust Jesus?" I lay there staring at her and I replied "Yes. Yes I trust Jesus." At last I found hope in the darkness. I was in a bad place but there was hope. I knew of a higher power and I was willing to trust him. Despite having been angry and feeling he was gone I knew he was there, and I was going to need him to get through this. No matter what happened I was going to leave it in God's hands and let him lead.

CHAPTER 2

Battling Leukemia and More

I knew I was in for the fight of my life. There had to be a way to get through this and I knew that it was going to take a lot of support and help. We started the task of telling everyone about what was going on and how they could help us. My mom and sister went to the oncologist office with us for our first visit. I wanted to make sure we didn't miss anything. They were there for moral support and to help us remember any and all questions we wanted to ask. Thankfully I had an amazing oncologist and their office and staff is the greatest and friendliest group of people on the face of the planet.

He didn't mind at all. He took the time to answer all of our questions. He explained how my cancer worked and that to start out I wouldn't have to go through any chemotherapy or radiation. They were going to put me on a regiment of Gleevec. It was a fairly new drug but they were having remarkable success with it. I said I would do whatever was necessary and that he wouldn't find a more model patient. It was at this time that I found one of my favorite verses **Philippians 4:6** *do not be* *anxious about anything, but in everything by prayer and supplication with thanksgiving let your requests be made known to God.* This single verse has brought me more peace than any other. I knew I had to let my nerves go and thank God for everything and learn from it.

It wasn't always easy though. Often those nerves would get the best of me. I remember days when my emotions were so messed up that I would sit and cry. I would shake and rock. I can honestly say that this was the darkest place that I had ever been in. Sometimes I didn't want to get out of bed. I hurt emotionally and I can honestly say that the emotional pain was much worse than any physical pain I could ever feel. Life was going around and around so quickly and I had no particular direction. I wanted to just get off the merry-go-round. I couldn't take it anymore. I was so thankful that my pastor took the time to come and visit with me and that my wife was so understanding. They lifted me up and carried me when I didn't have the strength to stand on my own. The stress and anxiety were running my life and they were slowly helping me to gain control of it back.

I knew that I had to let go of the anxiety and stress because they were only going to complicate matters. The road that lay ahead was going to be tough and I needed to work to make it as smooth as possible. So I set out with the mindset that I would be the best I could and always listen to the doctor. He wasn't going to be able to find a better behaved patient than I was going to be. His office started out wanting me off work for a full year so that they could get the medication levels straightened out. Here's where the next problem begin.

I went in to work and explained everything and despite the fact that I was on my laptop emailing and updating them from the hospital bed they were none too happy with the diagnosis and recommended time off. I filed the Family Medical Leave Act paperwork and my Disability paperwork for my short term disability. I notified work constantly of what was going on and kept them in the loop every step of the way. I even volunteered to work on my own time in order to help out so that they would not fall too far behind. My area vice president even commented that I completed more work in four hours from home than most people did in a full eight hour day at the office, but my immediate supervisor didn't see it that way. She didn't like me being out and she was dead set against holding my job.

I constantly did what I could to make sure not to lose my job but finally one day in November of 2008 I received a call and was told that I needed to come in to have a meeting with them. I had a feeling that this was not going to bode well for me. My anxiety was already high as I had been having severe headaches and I felt like I was probably losing my job. When I got there I found out that I was right. My supervisor said she could no longer hold my position if I was unable to return. The vice president then notified me that they had received authorization to create a work from home position for me once I returned. I would be able to work at my leisure as long as I pulled 40 hours a week, and they would work with me on appointments and things so that I would not have to worry about things. I was thrilled. I thought my prayers had been answered. Shortly thereafter I went into remission and I called my employer to let them know.

After much cajoling and promising not to overdo it the doctor agreed to let me return to work after the first of the year, this was only six months into the original year off they had wanted. The supervisor was thrilled and said she would get everything set up. Come the first of the year I called and she said they were not ready and that I was going to have to wait. So I waited. Then I got a call from my pastor and he wanted me to go to a conference with him in Indianapolis. I told him let me double check with my boss to make sure they did not want me to come in yet. The minute I told her about his offer she said she wanted me to return to work. So we set it up for me to come in that Monday morning and pickup my laptop and start training on my new duties. I was really bummed about not going, but I must say it was nice going back to work.

I thought finally things are looking up. I mean yes we were behind on bills, but I was in remission and returning to work so it wouldn't take long to get back on track. I got to the office and there was no laptop. They weren't even planning on me returning for another week or two; you can imagine that I was pretty upset at this point. I missed an opportunity to go to that conference for nothing and that didn't sit well with me. After I had been there for about an hour my supervisor ask me to come into her office to talk. It was then that she dropped the big bomb. My new job would not be work from home, my status was being changed so I was losing four vacation days, and I was being shifted to an hourly employee instead of a salaried employee. Because of my illness I was being demoted and discriminated against. I hit a major wall. Not only was I furious I was depressed, because I knew I was trapped between a rock and a hard place.

The problem was I had no choice but to accept her terms, because I needed a job and the insurance that went with it. Needless to say the doctor was not happy but since I was in remission there wasn't much we could do about it. So I settled in and took to learning my new duties. Within just about a month and half things begin to go downhill. The headaches started to return. I found myself tired all the time. I was sick more often than not. Working was slowly killing me. Rushing back to work was causing my leukemia to flare up and I was going downhill quickly.

I did the best I could but my illness was getting the best of me. I ended up seeing a neurologist for the headaches. The oncologist felt that the headaches were not related to the leukemia despite the fact that they were there when I first got sick and now that I was having trouble they were flaring up again. I went through six MRI's and two cat scans and numerous x-rays. The only thing they found was a small cyst in my sinus cavity nothing that would cause the intense debilitating headaches that I was experiencing. The first neurologist said that they were migraines associated with the leukemia. We tried many different medications and finally I found some relief, but then I started to pass blood through my bowels. The complications just kept coming.

I called the neurologist's office and they never called back. I talked to the oncologist and he said I should talk to the family doctor because he still did not think the headaches were related. I went to the family doctor and of course that warranted a colonoscopy. The colonoscopy turned up nothing. The blood work from the oncologist's office came back and I was no longer in remission, and the headaches were back with a vengeance. It couldn't get any worse, or so I thought. Unfortunately I was running out of vacation time and sick time. I was doing my best to keep my employer in the loop but I went in one day and received an e-mail to meet my supervisor in the vice-president's office in five minutes. I knew what was coming.

Earlier that morning I had informed my supervisor that I had two doctor's appointments later in the week and she said that it was no big deal that I could come in early and work around them, when I got to the vice-president's office that had all changed. They informed me that I had three options. Number one work the rest of the year and miss absolutely no time and need no schedule changes and I would keep my job. Number two continue to work and the next time I missed they would fire me unconditionally and fight any chance of unemployment. Lastly they offered a mutual agreement in which I would leave and they would provide me one month's wages and benefits. I had no choice. I took option three and finished the day and left on July 21, 2009 with that added stress on me.

I was out of work, getting sicker, and my insurance was going to run out real soon. My stress level was through the roof. The headaches were maxing out now. I spent many days in my bedroom in darkness with ice packs on my head taking pain medication trying to get some relief. My family doctor referred me to a neurologist in downtown Cincinnati. He was one of the best and he was also known for working with the Mayo clinic. The thing with this doctor was you had to send all of the information and your records, he would review them, and he would decide if he would take your case. I was hoping I would finally get some relief.

The oncologist upped my Gleevec dose to 600mg per day. We were going to try that to see if it would work rather than any other drastic measures. At least for now I wouldn't have to go through another bone marrow test or worse. The new neurologist called and they agreed to see me. They reviewed my records and he felt that there was something there. I filled out several pieces of paperwork. He finally decided on a drug regimen to treat the migraines and he felt that I needed to be treated for depression as well. He referred me to an ENT to test for food allergies, I also had to undergo physical therapy to relieve the strain that the stress was placing on my muscles, and he sent me to see a psychiatrist to learn some relaxation techniques. More doctors, more medicines and insurance running out. I had no clue what I was going to do but I had to try or I felt for sure I was going to go crazy.

I started the medications I was now up to 18 pills a day but I was willing to try and I set up the ENT appointment they did the blood work for the allergy testing. I was amazed at all the foods I was allergic to as well as other things such as trees, dust, weeds, and grass. I had to work on my eating habits and started the physical therapy. I was undergoing many treatments and exercises and the longer I was away from my job the better things got. The therapist felt that the constant staring at the computer might be contributing to the headache problems. He suggested that I should start focusing more on the things I love outdoors and relaxing and stay away from the computer more.

I needed to follow his directions, taking the medication, and going fishing to relax and I begin to improve. I was willing to do what it took. Finally I got the call from the oncologist's office I was back in remission. Maybe things were about to turn around. The headaches were getting better, I was in remission, and for the first time in a long time I was feeling pretty decent. My confidence was back and I was sure things were on the right track and I would be back on my feet in no time. Now to find a job and get back in the saddle!

CHAPTER 3

U-Turn

Things were looking up. I went to the Ohio State Firefighter's Conference and had a great time. I graduated from Indiana Wesleyan University on August 8, 2009 with a Bachelor's degree in Business Management and a Certificate in Religious Studies. I had no doubts that I would find a job and we would be cruising in no time. My studies with my pastor for my ministerial work were going well and I took the job as teacher of the Mixed Adults Sunday school class.

I begin to get my mojo back. The Sunday school class began to grow. The pastor's wife, Doodle, and her friend, Cathy, two members of my class stepped up and took the role of fun committee for the class. We started having breakfast during class and having special activities for fellowship and the response was amazing. I received a lot of good feedback about the teaching and this just encouraged me to keep going.

The unemployment was finally coming in, although there was a small snag, due to my company reporting health issues. The unemployment felt I should be on disability and disability said since I was in remission that I did not qualify. We got it straightened out and the checks were coming in, I was able to focus on finding that job. I got my resume all worked out and lined out and felt that it looked pretty good. I posted it on several career sites and was working very hard on finding a job.

Shortly thereafter I found out that my old company had a mass lay-off and I felt that God had given me a head start on finding a job. Several recruiters contacted me and they were impressed with my resume, and I got several hits from the job sites. I felt that it was just a matter of time. But the recession hit hard and the recruiters were having trouble finding anything and many of the independent contacts turned out to be scams. I would show up and they were group interviews with scam insurance companies or pyramid schemes. Many of these people even asking you to pay to come to the interview. As the time continued to drag on my desperation and depression begin to grow.

I started concentrating on the bills and the finances. I didn't have the ability to leave it in God's hands. I kept telling myself that I had to figure this out. As time marched on my stress level climbed. I felt so helpless and hopeless. The more I focused on my situation the less I focused on God. Every day became a struggle. Most of the time I didn't even want to get out of bed. Darkness was filling my heart and my mind. I saw no way out. Slowly but surely I was sinking into a bottomless pit of despair and heartache. No one really knew except maybe my wife. I was very good at hiding my feelings. I wasn't about to let anyone know that I was hurting. I was a man's man. I had to be strong and stay vibrant and active, but soon I was struggling to stand at all.

With each passing day it seemed that my life's blood was being sucked out of me. It was as if a vampire was sucking the very blood out of my body. My strength was waning, my heart was breaking, and I couldn't remember how to smile anymore. Life seemed pointless. Prayers became routine recitations and worship became empty void presentations for the benefit of those who were watching. I was ready to quit and simply lie down and die.

The U-turn was complete. I went from looking up to looking down. My confidence turned to pessimism. Happiness left me and sadness embraced me. I was grumpy, downtrodden, and broken. I begin to think about death a lot. Once again I felt that my family might be better off if I was gone. I even thought about ways to commit suicide to make it look like an accident. My insurance would only refund premiums if I committed suicide, so I had to make it appear as an accident to take care of my family.

I thought of poisons, running off a steep embankment and hoping to die in the fall, or a car accident. I was convinced the car accident was the best way to go. Of course then thoughts of failure entered my head and I kept picturing myself in a wheelchair. I would be a greater burden to my family than I was now. I was a coward. I couldn't do anything right. I was full of fear and dread. Every day was filled with sorrow and pain. I cried continually. I wasn't sleeping and the emotional toll was beginning to take a physical toll as well.

I would get the shakes, I was sick often, and the headaches were returning with some regularity and extreme severity. I was very nauseous and begin having stomach problems. I was weak and tired all the time. Rock bottom was my location and I had hit it very, very hard. There was no way out. The light had grown dim and only darkness remained. I was lost and wandering in the wilderness that was my life. I was being disobedient to God, I wasn't being a good father or husband, and friendship and family were being forsaken for self-pity and doubt. Only death held any appeal for me. The things of darkness held more attraction for me.

Just as Peter took his eyes off of Christ when he stepped out of the boat in **Matthew 14:29-31** *He said, "Come." So Peter got out of the boat and walked on the water and came to Jesus. But when he saw the wind, he was afraid, and beginning to sink he cried out, "Lord, save me." Jesus* *immediately reached out his hand and took hold of him, saying to him, "O you of little faith, why did you doubt?"* I had now taken my eyes off of Christ. Doubt and fear overwhelmed me and the more they grew, the less I listened for the voice of Jesus. The Spirit became a stranger to me. I could not recognize it because I did not want to face it. I knew I needed to turn back to the Lord. I knew I needed to be praying. And I knew I needed to pick myself up, but I didn't know how.

In my mind and opinion I was alone. To me no one could understand what I was going through or what I was facing. There wasn't anyone to help me and I had no encouragement or help to lift me out of the pit of shame and anger that I was digging. I hated the world. I didn't want sympathy, I didn't want pity, I just wanted it all to disappear and go away. I was going to focus on me and nothing else. I figured if I focused on myself and brought myself some pleasure then I would feel better and be able to rise up and be good again. I was going to fix me. I didn't need God. I didn't need religion. I could do it and I would show the world how valuable and how worthy I was. Notice in my darkest hour I sure didn't find any humility. I was being puffed up and I was going in circles on a rollercoaster I couldn't control.

CHAPTER 4

Escape & Visitation

They always say it's lonely at the top, but let me tell you it feels pretty lonely at the bottom as well. When life gets you down it intends to keep you there. You stop listening to people. Sure you hear them speaking but in all reality you have them half tuned out because you are so focused on fixing things yourself. I felt like there was nobody that cared and I had to face the terror and darkness alone.

I knew suicide wasn't the answer. I could never do that to my wife and kids. I loved them way too much to hurt them like that. I have seen the pain and heartache that such an act can cause. So to get away I begin to read and watch TV like a madman. When I say I was reading I mean I was doing some serious reading. I would read a 300 page book in just a couple of hours. I used the book as an escape.

I wasn't just reading I was traveling into the story. I would become a part of the novel. I would build false realities around the story and the characters I was reading about. I used this to strengthen myself and to find solace and comfort. Instead of going to God and the Bible, I ran to suspense novels with tales of murder, spies, and evil. These books become a way for me to escape the pain, because in the story I could be the hero. I could be everything I wasn't being in real life. Fantasy was more fun than real life. So I begin spending more time there, than I did inside my miserable life.

My wife would volunteer at school with our boys so I would be left at home all alone. I would flip on the television and find ghost hunting shows, or shows about haunting, sometimes it was just violent crime shows. I became a junky I would watch these for hours on end. Then I would lie awake at night, my mind going a hundred miles an hour replaying the evil that I had taken in earlier that day. Insomnia became commonplace and I begin to sleep half the day and watch garbage TV all night.

Now at this time I need to make a few confessions. First like most people I have some natural fears in life. No I am not afraid of snakes or spiders. I am not claustrophobic; however I am terrified of heights and darkness. I do not know why. I have learned to deal with both of my fears, but sometimes they still can shake me. I remember growing up as a child I would lie in bed and listen to every sound. I was always sure that someone was coming to get me. I heard every dog bark, every tree branch snap, and every owl screech.

Every sound to me was an ominous sign of evil coming to get me. I would dream of monsters and demons tormenting me. One terrible dream I had particular was that I would be sleeping on the couch and it was dark, I would look at the door, and peering in was a ghastly white face. The door knob would turn and in would come this hideous man who was going to kill me and my family. I would try to scream but I was so afraid that no sound would come. So there I would sit trembling, crying, he would raise his knife and strike. And I would awake. Shaking, sweating, and scared to death.

Now as an adult I know that the dark is just that and I can go outside in the dark, and I can walk around my house at night. But even today sometimes if the mood is poor enough my anxiety can make me nervous and shaky especially in unfamiliar areas or in troubling times. So here I was severely depressed, embracing fantasy more than reality, turning away from God, and watching and reading about the satanic, evil, and wicked. I was in the darkness and my fear went into hyper-drive.

As I watched a particular series call "The Haunting" my mind began to race. The evil begin to encroach and I couldn't stop it anymore. The shows begin to run together in my mind. I would lie awake and see demons in my home, I was hearing voices and sounds, and the ghosts were around every corner. I didn't want to be left alone in my own home. I didn't even want to close my eyes, because I knew the monsters would be there. In all honesty I had lost it. I was losing my mind and I had lost control. The battle inside me was raging. Finally one night it came to a head.

I went to bed that night and actually fell asleep. Then the dream or vision started. The voice called out to me, and told me that I would never be any good for God and that I was going to be useless and that the time for me to die had come. **Ephesians 6:12** *For we do not wrestle against flesh and blood, but against the rulers, against the authorities, against the cosmic powers over this present darkness, against the spiritual forces of evil in the heavenly places,* was all too real to me now. In my dream this horribly disfigured demon came to me and he grabbed me and told me he was dragging me into hell so that I could not be of any service to God. He started to pull and scream. It was the worst thing I have ever seen or heard. But he couldn't pull me down because something had a hold of me. I looked back and there was my pastor, his wife, and my wife holding on to me pulling me back. They were re-assuring me and encouraging me to fight and to hold on. I begin to pull away from the demon and they finally pulled me free. At this point my wife woke me up, because I was thrashing about in the bed and screaming in my sleep.

I have no doubt that Satan was trying to stop me from working for God at this time. He used my circumstances to push me down lower, and he tried to take me out of service permanently. I am positive that the demon in my dream was real that night. I am also certain that it was love that saved me. The love of friends, family, and of God that preserved me on that dreadful night.

My depression had weakened me emotionally and physically. My pride had weakened me spiritually. My stubbornness had weakened my devotion, and my selfishness had weakened my resolve. When all this was coupled together my vision was blurred. I took my eyes off of Jesus and I looked to myself for strength and what I found was sin and wickedness. I invited the devil in and he accepted readily and heartily. I had to get right with God and I did. I realized that I had many family and friends I could count on and turn to but I had to put my pride aside. God had taught me a very valuable lesson.

I made a vow that I would not watch those kinds of shows anymore. I took greater care in what I watched and what I listened to. I begin to talk to people more about how I felt and what I was facing. I picked up my Bible and other Godly reading materials. I got a re-alignment. The car was now running a little straighter and the shimmy was gone. The terrible car wreck that was my life was now running smooth and straight once again. I started praying again and the funk began to fade. I found a new purpose. It was at this time that I was called to teach and with this new purpose and motivation I started to grow closer to God. I received my next visitation this time from the Holy Spirit.

As I studied and read I begin to notice so many new things. I was watching Christian shows, reading Christian books, and listening to Christian music and podcasts. One day I was jamming out to some Christian music and I remember this awesome presence just engrossed me. And I heard a voice say to me. "I know it has been hard, but I still love you and you are valuable and have a special purpose. Don't ever forget that." I was so overwhelmed I was crying big crocodile tears. I had never felt so uplifted and so vibrant in all my life. I knew from that moment on no matter how despairing or low I might get, I would never lose hope again.

Life is worth living. Live it well. We are always in such a hurry that we don't slow down and enjoy the moment, but believe you me. When you escape after having the visits I have had you find a new appreciation for life. Does this mean life suddenly got terrific and everything was great? Of course not, I still had many difficulties and struggles and we will look at those and the differences now that I had learned to rely on God instead of myself.

CHAPTER 5

The Encouragers

In all things life is easier when you have help. God knew this, which is why in the beginning he created Eve for Adam. The Bible tells us in **Genesis 2:18** *Then the LORD God said, "It is not good that the man should be alone; I will make him a helper fit for him.* People need companionship. We need that special someone who is there when we need them and who is like us, and cares for us, and is willing to help us. Alone is never a good place to be. We are more susceptible when we are alone. That is why the darkness and evil were able to get me so easily because I had alienated myself and was alone. I tried to go it alone and found that I needed help and support.

Ask any manager or supervisor the key to running a successful business or office and they will tell you it is the support structure. Ask any contractor the key to having a sturdy building is a strong support structure. The same holds true for our Christian life. We need a strong support structure to help us through the tough times and to lift us up out of the pit of despair. You need people who will share your burdens, people who will teach you, and people who will encourage you through their example.

My first encourager is easy for me to name and that is my wife, Tori. No matter what my circumstances she has always been there for me. She loves me unconditionally. Here I am sick, out of work, not providing, not being loving, disconnected, and plain and simply being mean sometimes; yet she would love on me, hug me, kiss me and tell me it's going to be okay. She always said as long as we have each other that's all we need. She helped me find God after my diagnosis, and she helped to lift me out of my depression. When I teach I ask her for feedback, I bounce ideas off her for my sermons and get more feedback, and she listens when I need to vent. No matter what I decide or choose to do she is right there supporting me 100 percent. When I say I can't she says I can. When I give up she helps me go again. And when I need to slow down she hits the brakes. I am truly blessed that God created her for me.

Next would have to be my pastor, Chad Blevins. He has helped to tutor me in the Bible. He has counseled with me when I needed to talk. He visited me when I was sick and depressed. He encouraged me in my preaching and teaching. He is a shining example of someone who loves and cares about giving and about missions. Reaching the world is truly his goal. He reminds me so much of Barnabas in the Bible. I think about **Acts 4: 32-37**

Now the full number of those who believed were of one heart and soul, and no one said that any of the things that belonged to him was his own, but they had everything in common. And with great power the apostles were giving their testimony to the resurrection of the Lord Jesus, and great grace was upon them all. There was not a needy person among them, for as many as were owners of lands or houses sold them and brought the proceeds of what was sold and laid it at the apostles' feet, and it was distributed to each as any had need. Thus Joseph, who was also, called by the apostles Barnabas (which means son of encouragement), a Levite, a native of Cyprus, sold a field that belonged to him and brought the money and laid it at the apostles' feet. That would be my pastor, willing to give it all for others; encouraging and lifting people up, always finding the best in people and bringing unity and peace by meeting their needs. I am truly honored and blessed to have a mentor like him.

Next would be my family, my mom and dad, my sister, and brother. I grew up in a non-Christian home, but it was a home filled with love and respect. I learned so much about loyalty and family devotion that it gave me a foundation to live my life upon. My mom has stood with me through thick and thin. Like I said earlier my mom and my sister went to the oncologist with me. If I need something I know I can call them. I know they are there. That's what family is about and what we stand for. My mom and I talk almost every day and even today she knows where I am most of the time.

When my wife and I are out and about my mom still knows. We visit regularly and we confide often. My dad never spoke much and is not an emotional person, but he is a rock. I know he cares and he is the foundation of our family. I am so proud to carry his name, and pray that I will always make him proud and bring honor to our family.

After them would be my former Sunday school teacher, Don Larrison. He is also my deacon but no one has shown more faith and trust in me than he has. He has always been there with kind words, love and affection, and encouragement. He is the kindest and most compassionate man I have ever met. My wife refers to him as Cottontop, because he has white hair. It is a term of endearment to her for him. He is everyone's grandpa. When people are hurting and in need he gives, when people are sick he visits, and when I have to miss class he teaches. He supports the church in so many ways as well as the community. He is not ashamed of his faith and he inspires me to be proud of my own faith. He is my hero of the faith.

Next would be the pastor's wife and a good friend of hers who are in my Sunday school class. My pastor's wife has a nickname and it is Doodle. I love it. She is real. She loves baseball, she is a teacher, and she is extremely knowledgeable when it comes to the Bible. She helps with tough topics in class and her friend, Kathy, stepped up and volunteered to be the fun committee for my class. They plan many events such as breakfast, going to a hockey game, a game night, a cook out, and even a white water rafting trip to Gatlinburg. They have been a blessing to me and to the class, and they encourage me so much by their examples.

These are just a few there are many, many more like my in-laws they have been there for me more times than I can count. They have taught me compassion, patience, and how to be laid back; also my mother-in-law is blind but she has not allowed that to slow her down. She still serves the Lord and stays active in the community. She is an inspiration to everyone who knows her. I also have a new gentleman in my class who is a former school superintendent. He has fought many personal battles and he is amazingly intelligent. He also fills in sometimes when I am out. He is such an example just by the way he conducts and carries himself and I look forward to growing closer to him and being mentored by him. Lastly is another pastor friend of mine, Ben, who has given me some opportunities to preach. He has been there to counsel with me and to encourage me. I appreciate his support and love very much. He is good Godly man and I look forward to a long and bountiful relationship between him and me and both our churches. The key is I have a great support network. The problem was I didn't know enough to use it and didn't tap into it when I needed it. I can assure you I will never make that mistake again. What good is a support structure if you don't use it?

The main support though will always be my grandfather. My "pappy" was an amazing man. He never met a stranger. He was a friend to everyone and loved the Lord. Church was a passion for my grandfather and he took me all the time as a child. Some of my fondest memories are the times I spent with him sitting under the old hedge row, while he tinkered with old lawn mowers or working in his garden. Sundays were always the Lord's day and he would spend it at church or reading his Bible. He inspires me to serve God and I will always cherish him. He has gone on to be with the Lord now and I pray that he will always be in the forefront of my heart and mind as I serve in my ministry.

One thing I have learned is that there are many people who care about me, and I assure you there are many people who care about you as well. I am extremely fortunate because I belong to a very loving church. Nothing can take the place of a loving church. They will give you support, encouragement, and love no matter what you face. When you are down they will pick you up. They will share your burdens and ease your cares. They can also help you to find uplifting and refreshing worship. The Bible tells us that **Matthew 18:20** *For where two or three are gathered in my name, there am I among them."* There is power in fellowship with our Christian brothers and sisters. So many times I have gone to church feeling down and I leave feeling renewed and excited, all because I enjoyed fellowship with the encouragement of my brothers and sisters in the Lord. It's all part of the support. There are many blessings found in having the proper support in place.

Work with your family. Rebuild and renew relationships. Communicate with your family they are a great source of refreshing and companionship. Be upfront with your church, you will be amazed at the love and support you will find. If you don't have a church, find one. Get into your local church, and get active and find the love and fellowship that it can give you. All too often the support structure is there, we simply don't know how to assemble it and access it.

CHAPTER 6

Cruise Control

For the time being I felt like control and sanity had been restored. There would be no more down spells. It was time to take control and get back in the game. I was ready to be a rock star! God is good and He was in control. At last I had found peace and comfort in who I was and how things were going. I was not scared, nervous, or worried like I had been before. The cruise control was set and I was flying down the highway.

Things actually went quite well for some time. I was able to get the bills caught up. We paid off all of our credit debt. School was going very well. My Sunday school class was growing and the teaching was going well. I had several opportunities to preach and my ministry seemed to be growing and I felt like I was growing as a Christian.

One of the highlights of this period was the opportunity to start attending some meetings with my pastor. These were the Southern Hills Baptist

Association meetings. This is an organization of Baptist churches who work cooperatively as members of the Southern Baptist Convention. I met several people and begin to network some and decided to take a class on the Book of Acts through the Seminary Extension program that they offered at the Association office. It was in this class that a met a couple of good leaders and begin to develop my desire to learn and study more of the Bible.

The teacher for the class was a pastor of one of the member churches and he was a very godly man. His name was Tim Cline and he taught me a great deal about being a Christian and a leader of a church. I can never say enough about the wisdom he passed on to me in that class and I will forever be in his debt for sharing his knowledge and guidance.

The other man I met was Ben Hurst. Brother Ben was then and has continued to be an extremely close friend, encourager, supporter, and mentor. Outside of my pastor, Ben has been one of my closest allies in the faith. We developed a great friendship during our class together, many nights after class standing in the parking lot talking for an hour or more. So many times we just get lost in conversation.

Ben has given me multiple opportunities to fill in at his church to preach. I have enjoyed his encouragement and feedback. His church has been a real blessing to both me and my wife. They embrace us and make us feel extremely welcome. I have also been fortunate enough to preach at the Relay for Life event in Eastgate, Ohio. This is a fund raising event to benefit cancer research and has been a great way for me to work for a great cause, share my faith, and to share my fight with cancer. God was using everything and blessing me mightily.

I begin teaching the men's group at church and my Sunday school class took a trip to Gatlinburg, TN for a whitewater rafting trip. Life was good. My family had learned to live on less but enjoy life more. The simple things brought us greater pleasure and the world no longer held the allure that it once did. Everything was going well. For the first time I felt the hope, the confidence, and the joy that I knew I should have as a Christian.

I started sending applications out to many different churches across the country and still applying to different positions online, so it was just a matter of time before a job popped up. There was never a chance, in my mind, that my time on unemployment would last very long. I was so very wrong. I begin to get turn down notices from churches, no responses or hits on my resume, the interviews were few and far between. The days turned into weeks, and the weeks turned into months. If it had not been for the federal extended benefits I am not sure what I would have done. My cruise control was broken and I was on an uphill climb and losing all momentum fast.

I tried to stay in my primary field of insurance but what few interviews I could find were with scams or group interviews which turned out to be jokes. Often some of them even wanted money up front to continue in the interview process! I expanded my field and tried searching many avenues and I did get a few bites but it always seemed that when the topic of the mutual agreement to leave my previous employer came up I was in trouble. They would ask me to explain and I would tell them it was based on a medical issue and sometimes I even explained the Leukemia and how I was in remission and able to do whatever, but it didn't matter, the interview soon ended and I never heard from them again.

I was floundering and there seemed to be nothing I could do. I was teaching, studying, attending seminary, praying, attending church doing everything I knew to do to try to get God to help me, yet it seemed that no matter what I was destined to failure and misery. Everything I touched turned to tragedy and pain. I was a complete and total failure. I couldn't find a job. I couldn't support my family. I couldn't be a real man and take of the responsibilities that I had here on Earth. Cruise control was off and the brakes had been heavily applied. My depression started to climb again and I knew that it wasn't going to be long before I would be in a very bad place. Why wasn't God listening to me? Why was he letting me struggle so much? How could he hate me this much and what did I do to deserve all of this? I was Job losing everything and my friends were even there to dig at me.

It didn't take long that I heard rumors that people questioned whether or not I was really looking for a job or if I knew how to fill out an application. I was stunned and shocked! The economy stunk, we were in the Great Recession as they were calling it, and unemployment was at an all-time high. I was a college graduate with a management degree and I finished with high honors, yet the people who supposedly knew me and cared for me questioned my ability and desire to work. Talk about getting slapped in the face! I was angry, hurt, and disgusted. It wasn't long before I was ready to leave the church for greener pastures, if I had only known where they could be found.

CHAPTER 7

Struggling to be disciplined

My feelings were hurt and I felt like the church wasn't my home anymore. I begin to see every flaw in every person and process of the church. Before I knew it I was ready to snap. I was allowing my anger to become malicious and controlling. The wheels in my head were spinning around and around, and I was finding it more and more difficult to focus on anything spiritual. All of the anger that was burning inside was directed toward the church, toward the deacons, toward my pastor, and toward my family. In all reality no one was safe the world was the target, Satan was pulling the trigger, and I was willingly serving as the sniper! My emotions were in control and they were in total submission to my worldly and fleshly attitude.

I knew I was out of God's will, and I knew that there was no way out of the darkness that I found myself in. The problem was that I was allowing my anger control me, not my sense, or my spirit. Life was eating me up and I had no clue how to escape the cycle I was going through. Every night when I lay down to go to bed I would sit there unable to sleep; my mind would just race with anxiety and frustration. I was irritated and the more I looked at things the more problems I could find. I found myself nitpicking everything. I would sit and complain and moan about everything. Happiness avoided me and there was no joy to be found anywhere in my soul. I focused on the sorrow, the pain, and the failures in my life. I was as pessimistic as it could get.

The first target of my anger was the financial committee at my church. There were things I felt needed to be done and I felt that we needed to do some modernizing of the facilities and our service. Whenever something wasn't done or didn't get approved I would become so angry. One major issue we argued over was a copy machine. I thought that machine needed to be replaced and they felt it was fine. The church had budgeted the money but it turned into an ugly fight to get it. In one of the business meetings I lost my temper and actually smarted off to one of the deacons, who was also on the committee. I was ready to explode.

This is just one example of the way my mind was attacking people around me. I was not a nice person to be around. So when I would go to church I usually came home complaining about something. I was not being blessed, because I was not really attending. I was merely present. I was disciplined in attending and that was about it. My heart was not fully present. The problem with this is that when you are like that you get really hardened. You begin to lose your empathy, your sympathy, your caring, and your love.

First I begin to stop studying, then I stopped reading, and then I stopped praying the way I should. I turned my back on the things of God. I struggled to stay disciplined. I was spiraling down into a dark world of sin. Open rebellion against the things of God and worrying only about myself and my carnal desires. There was no quiet time, no meditation, and no devotion. This is how I not only got lost in the dark, but how I eagerly, greedily, and earnestly ran into sin. I gave into my envy, greed, coveting, jealousy, anger, rage, materialism, self-loathing, selfishness, and pride. In the famous words of "Star Wars", I went over to the dark side.

In my opinion reading was boring, God's word was too convicting for me to read. I was out of meeting with my pastor on a regular basis, and thus I had no accountability. When you are out of God's word it becomes very easy to look for fulfillment and satisfaction in anything else. The television became my friend; I spent hours on end watching the "idiot" box. I loved to read, but there were no books that I enjoyed anymore. I was walking away from who I was. The devil had a grip on me and his main goal was to pull me away from God and my church family.

Secondly was stopping the prayer and meditation. Bottom line is when you don't talk to

God then you never receive the renewal of his Spirit that helps to refresh and invigorate you. This leaves you all alone against the powers of darkness that come against you to assail you at every turn. Trust me when I say in the darkness and against the powers of evil, alone is the one thing that you do not want to be. When I had ended up trapped in watching the shows that revolved around the supernatural, I was alienated from my church, from my friends, and from my family. I was alone! I had abandoned all the things that helped me to stay true to God's word. I was without God, without his word, and without his uplifting renewal. Without discipline I had fallen into mediocrity and sin.

Just like anything on Earth, any sport, any business, and any organization there are certain disciplines that help people rise above and to be the best at what they do. It takes practice, it takes exercise, it takes experience, and it takes hard work and dedication. Our Christian life is no different. I had tried to go on cruise control and I lost my discipline and this let me fall into a life that was not only displeasing to God, but it was dishonoring to my church, embarrassing to my family, and degrading to my spirit. I was struggling to be disciplined and it was killing me as a Christian.

Chapter 8

The Awakening

Now you may have noticed that there was something missing in the last two chapters. There were no Bible verses present in those chapters. This was an intentional omission to represent the lack of God's presence in my life during the darkest times and trials. I had no semblance of religion and Christianity in me and this was a major problem. Thankfully the simple act of attendance kept me in the presence of God, his word, and his people enough to allow him to work in my life without my permission or submission.

I was hurting, I felt lonely, and I was simply struggling. I felt like my ministry wasn't growing, my class was suffering, and my men's group was just not growing. In plain terms I felt like a total failure. I was unemployed, my ministry was failing, and my life was without meaning. There were more days of gloom and doom than anything else in my life. I wanted to sleep all the time, I barely had enough energy to get off the couch and pick up the house a little bit, and commitments became a scary item that I just did not want to do. Depression seemed to grow all around me and was readily embraced by my carnal self.

There were many days where I wanted to give up all of my teaching and leadership positions, sometimes just going to church was a chore, and my creative inspirational side was floundering on the shore of "woe is me" and the "why me?" sea. Often I would sit teary eyed and lost in confusion and desperation. By the grace of God, my wife kept me teaching, kept me attending, and God sent all of the Barnabus Christians I needed. My dear friend Floyd would talk to me at church and always encourage me and he shared with me how the men's meetings had helped him through difficult struggles. One of my favorite people in the world, whom I admire as a person and as a Christian, Kathy told me how much my teaching in Sunday school had helped her. And many other students in my class shared out of the blue what I meant to them as their teacher: Ruth said "she learned more than all of years in another class", Brenda "thanked me for making the Bible understandable", Bill told me "You don't give yourself enough credit, and that you do a good job." My position as one of God's vessel was confirmed and I had to eat a lot of crow. God called me back into the fold that day so that I would be more flexible, more useful, more coherent, and more adaptable, but more importantly I would never doubt his ability to work in me again.

Now please do not misinterpret my new attitude. I am not saying any of this to be prideful or boastful, but I realized that I was so busy concentrating on me and feeling sorry for myself and what I didn't have or what I hadn't achieved that I was missing the miracles and blessings that God was performing right in front of my own eyes. I will never again doubt Him, I will never again ask why, and I will never again wonder if; but rather I will look for the open door, I will ask what do you want me to learn, where is the blessing, and how can I be a useful tool for God to use. Can I bring God glory through the trial, the darkness, and the persecution? I want my witness to sing of his providence, not abandonment. Will people see my joy, and not my sorrow? I pray that I will be an example, not a stumbling block.

My church family saved me from the pit of despair and I vowed to never let them down again. I know the value of the local church and the local congregation. Our fellow brothers and sisters help to shape us, they help to guide us, and they help to lift us up when we need it. I thought about two verses. The first verse is one that my friend Floyd quoted to me **Proverbs 27:17** *Iron sharpens iron, and one man sharpens another.* The people around us shape us and God helps us by putting the necessary people in our lives to sharpen us. We become better, our knowledge grows, our experience grows, our faith grows, and our Christian witness grows as well. By having men around me who loved me enough to talk to me about the things I was doing wrong and helping me to fix them so that I could grow as a Christian. Also the women of the church were there to help me to know that I can be more open and sharing and that it is okay to build relationships in a Christian manner.

This confirms the second verse and the value of fellowship, **Hebrews 10: 24-25** [24]*And let us consider how to stir up one another to love and good works,* [25] *not neglecting to meet together, as is the habit of some, but encouraging one another, and all the more as you see the Day drawing near.* If I had quit going to church all together I know without a doubt that I would have been lost to sin. I would have embraced all the more the world and its view of life and what it means to succeed and to be successful. Instead I found the truth of the scriptures, and that is the true frailty of mankind. We cannot be left to our own devices. Man is not trustworthy and we are not reliable. On our own we will FAIL! By ourselves we will stumble. Without fellowship, both with the church and with God, we are not disciplined and we are not faithful.

God understands this that is why he commands us to gather together. He knows our needs and our hearts. There is no question that when left to our own devices we will choose self and destruction that leads to self-destruction every time. No one wants to fail, no one wants to be responsible for their self-destruction, no one wants to be the blame, but the reality is that we are sinful beings and without God then we are rotten to the core. No matter how good we think we are, no matter how much good work we do, no matter how morally we live we are a disappointment in God's eyes and we are bound for hell. We are failures as his favored creation, because we are disobedient and contemptuous creatures who disregard his teachings and his guidance.

The problem is when this reality sets in it can destroy us. We can fall down, we can sink into depression, and then we begin to grasp with the reality of our carnality and our limitations. This is when we begin to doubt ourselves and our abilities. The fact remains that this is when God can use us the most, because He needs us to realize that we cannot do it of ourselves, it is only through his power that we live, breathe, and survive. This is where that need for fellowship comes in.

This is the reality that I awoke to. I woke up and realized that I had to stay connected to Christ. I had to listen to his music, I had to read his word, I had to hear his preaching and teaching, I had to talk to him and fellowship with his people. It was this reality that has inspired me to be stronger, more courageous, and bolder in my witnessing and testifying. I know that I have said that I could worship God without going to church. I said I could worship without listening to preaching and teaching. I said I didn't need fellowship to grow and live as a Christian. I was wrong! I needed my church family and I needed my connection with God. I was awake and it was time to put the pieces back together and make this puzzle that was my life, transform into the beautiful masterpiece that Christ wanted it to be. It was meant to be a testimony for him, a vessel through which his love could flow. It was not meant to be a broken jar shattered on the floor with all of the life giving water poured out on the ground, useless, and wasted.

Chapter 9

I Will Rise

Chapter eight I started out by saying that I had omitted Bible verses from chapters six and seven to represent the lack of God's presence in my life. After I had awakened I realized that God was not gone, his presence was still there, and as a matter of fact it was his presence that saved me from burrowing down into the depths of despair. God had shown me that I had to be cleansed in order to be used. **2 Timothy 2:20-22** *[20]Now in a great house there are not only vessels of gold and silver but also of wood and clay, some for honorable use, some for dishonorable. [21]Therefore, if anyone cleanses himself from what is dishonorable, he will be a vessel for honorable use, set apart as holy, useful to the master of the house, ready for every good work. [22]So flee youthful passions and pursue righteousness, faith, love, and peace, along with those who call on the Lord from a pure heart.* Life had now changed. I had experienced the salvation experience, but now I was experiencing the ministry call and God had shown me that I could rise above the world through his empowerment.

Now I am not saying that I don't have bad days. There are still tough days when my emotions are crazy and life is hard, but I now remember who is in control and I fully trust in that. I am more devoted to my teaching and preaching than ever. I listen to the Bible, I read the Bible, I study, I listen to good preaching, I attend church, I read Godly works, I fellowship with Christians, I turn off the world, I walk away from sin, I consciously choose my attitude and mood, but most importantly I pray, I meditate, I sacrifice, I give, I listen, I obey. Am I perfect? By no means and let me tell you I fall down on many occasions. I am not bragging, what I am doing is telling you that God was able to speak to my heart, He was able to transform my sinful nature to an obedient soul, and He was able to help me to rise from the ashes of my self-loathing and pitiful misery.

God showed me that He could raise me up and use me, when I was unable to do anything in my own strength and power. Chris Tomlin sings the song "I Will Rise" and this song really speaks to me, because it doesn't matter how bad things get today or in this world, I know that in eternity I will rise to live with Christ and that is the ultimate reward. No matter how bad it gets I have hope, I can endure, and I can overcome.

Sometimes in order to be useful we have to take the material we are using and start over from scratch. It is the same with us as humans, sometimes God has to tear us down and then build us back up into the useful tool that he can use to edify the church and spread the gospel. When times get tough, and life seems so unfair remember this simple fact. God uses those people that are BROKEN!

BROKEN

A Caregiver's View

By

VICTORIA L. TULL

You never forget the day when your job goes from being a wife to being a caregiver. You go from worrying about the everyday things like bills and the kids to having to keep track of doctor's appointments and medicines. I became the encourager and cheerleader even though I was falling apart inside.

For me that day came on June 18, 2008. It was the day that the doctor walked into Doug's hospital room and told us that he had Chronic Myelogenous Leukemia or CML.

The week started just like any other week. Doug was working, the kids were on summer break, and we were living on the farm. The kids went to my mother-in-law's house to stay the night, because we bought a couple of goats and we were picking them up and building the pen for them.

Even June 12th started like a normal day. Doug went to work and I got up and started making plans for the goats. I went down and picked the kids up and had them helping me set up everything for our newest additions to the farm. Then around 4 o'clock in the afternoon the phone rang, it was Doug and he had a fever and a major headache. He didn't think that he could drive so I made him a doctor's appointment and loaded up the kids and went to get him. When I got to him, he was complaining of a stiff neck and just to look at him I knew he was really sick.

We went straight to the doctor and by the time he was taken back, his fever was 104 degrees. The doctor sent him straight to the hospital and said he thought Doug might have Meningitis. On our way to the hospital I called my mother-in-law to meet us at the hospital to pick up the kids. I didn't know what was going to happen or how long we would be at the hospital.

Once we got to the ER they took him straight back and started taking blood and got things ready to do a spinal tap. Thankfully his mom got there at that point so I and the kids stepped out to go meet her. That way the kids wouldn't be in the room for the procedure. While I was outside the doctors tried three times to do a lumber puncture and didn't get it. When I came back in they decided to take him to x-ray to get it done.

About a half hour or so after we got there his blood work came back and showed his white blood count was over forty thousand and they decided to admit him into the hospital to run more tests. So then it became a hurry up and wait game. Hurry up to get the tests run and wait to get the results. They began testing him for everything under the sun. He was turned into a pin cushion because they would come in to take blood and take like six or seven pop bottles full. It was crazy.

At one point during the week they put him in quarantine which included me because I was staying with him. They made me wear a mask and everything anytime I stepped out of the room. I didn't leave him very much because I wasn't sure he would be alive when I came back. I started to mentally prepare myself to not only be a widow but also raise two boys on my own.

By this time his headaches were so bad that we couldn't turn the lights on so every time someone came to visit they were afraid to come in because they thought he was sleeping.

We celebrated Father's Day while he was in the hospital. My in-laws brought the boys down to see us and our biggest fear was whether or not they would get to see daddy for another Father's Day. The doctors were clueless at this point as to what was going on with Doug. They were doing all kinds of tests and procedures and everything seemed to come back okay. Only his white blood count was off. On Monday that week they decided to test his bone marrow to see what was going on there. They had to try twice to get the marrow because they didn't get enough the first time.

I cried a lot that week because of the not knowing what was going on, when or even if he was going to get out of the hospital and even if he would live. I cried because of how much pain he was in and because I couldn't do anything to help him. I felt like I was going to lose my best friend, and I was lost.

During the week that we were at the hospital a good friend of ours came in with her husband who had cancer. Bev Seale is a sweet woman who we knew through school and church and she became the person I leaned on. She was where I was going to be and knew how I felt. I truly feel like God put them there to help us get through this. She was there with us when we got test results and when the doctors had no idea where to go next.

We also had a great nighttime nurse that was amazing for me and Bev because she took care of our men so we could take a breath. She was even going to "babysit" the guys so we could go out and have a real meal. However, it never happened because Bev's husband George ended up having a procedure that took most of the day and so it was late and we were both tired. The night ended up good though because I went and got a couple of movies and we snuggled in his bed and watched movies on his laptop. It was nice to have some kind of normal again, even though he had IVs and monitors attached to him.

The morning of June 18th started out like normal but by the time it was over our world was flipped upside down. Dr. Ruehlman was the oncologist who was working on Doug's case and he came in that afternoon and told us that Doug had

CML. I was stunned he had leukemia, people die from leukemia. Was did this mean, was he going to die? But wait wasn't it only kids that got leukemia? Doug was in his thirties, so it couldn't be this. Could it?

When Dr. Ruehlman told us that he had this I couldn't say it so I asked him to write it down on a piece of paper. I comforted Doug for a couple of minutes after the doctor left, then I went out to the hallway and found our nurse and just held up the paper that said

Chronic Myelogenous Leukemia

and then I broke. The nurse went and got Bev and she read it and just hugged me and held me while I cried my heart out. I didn't know what to do but I knew I couldn't break in front of Doug, he was broken enough and I had to be strong.

Once I got myself together I went back into the room with Doug and held him while he cried then came the hardest part telling our family. We lost eight people that year several to cancer, so to tell our families that Doug had cancer was really hard to do. Everyone cried no one knew what else to do at that point. We spent the rest of the day telling people and not really knowing what else to do but cry.

The next day became a day of learning more. I woke up that morning deciding to learn as much about this and if and how to beat it. Doug was not going to die; I was going to do everything in my power to save him. I didn't care what it took; I was going to find help. So I began searching the internet pouring over anything I could find about CML. Dr. Ruehlman came in the next day and I had a ton of questions for him about this. What treatment options were there? Was there medicine he could take, if so what was it and how did we get it? This was cancer so did that mean chemo or radiation? If so, how soon could he start? What could he expect to be his quality of life, or how long could he live? I wanted to know everything and anything that could help.

Dr. Ruehlman was great he took this time to answer my questions. Like yes there was medicine, no, he didn't need chemo at this time and yes he could live a full long life. We found out that he was going to be started on Gleevec, an amazing pill that could put him and keep him in remission, however he would need to take it probably the rest of his life and it was expensive. I didn't care I was going to do everything I could to get this for him. And I had to fight to get it. The insurance wouldn't cover it if I got it from a pharmacy, I would have to do mail order to get it. But wait it could take up to a week to get it in, and he needed to start it now. So I fought with the insurance to get it covered once from the regular pharmacy and after that we would get it mail order, whatever we needed to do.

I started to breathe a little better once we got the medicine and he started taking it. I was still worried but at least we were going in the right direction.

It was hard to keep positive but I was going to do my best. I had Doug and the boys to think about, and I couldn't let them down. So I did what I do best, I hid and cried. When I was around anyone I was the strong, supportive go-getting wife, mother and caregiver. However, when I was alone I cried. I cried for the unknown, the fear, the anger, and the disbelief that this was happening.

I thought that we had our share of problems. You see we had a son with Autism, and my mom was blind and I thought nothing would happen because I wasn't strong enough to handle any more than that. I was shown that I was not in control of anything; God was in control of everything.

I remember when we were getting our oldest, Douglas, tested for autism. One of the tests that they did was an EEG where they attached the wires to his head, he was two at the time and they had to put him in a papoose to attach everything because he didn't like things around his head. One of the hardest parts of this procedure was when he looked up at us and cried, "Why, what do?" because

I knew this was going to be good for him but I couldn't change it at the time.

Fast forward six years and I wanted to cry to God, "Why, what do?" The good thing is that God knew that it would be a good thing for our family, but we needed this challenge to accept different changes in our life.

Things have changed a lot since he was diagnosed with CML. He has accepted the call to preach, we stopped taking things for granted. Family time and date nights became important parts to us because you never know when life will end. It's like the Tim McGraw song, live like you were dying. That is how we live life now. Why put off something that you really want to do, when you don't know if another chance will come.

A cancer diagnoses is something that turns your world upside down and can send you into a deep depression if you let it. Or you can look at it like a gift from God like we do and be thankful for every minute that you have together. All of the sudden the little fights and arguments seem like no big deal. You smile when you wake up and your husband is there and okay. You still cry sometimes at the not knowing but you smile when his blood tests come back and they are good and he is in remission. You celebrate the anniversary of the diagnoses date because it is another year that you get to have your best friend healthy.

For a long time I cried every time we went to the oncologist's office because I couldn't believe this was really our life. I was saddened to think that we were going through things that people went through when they were older. Weren't we too young for this? Let me tell you, a lot of people wonder the same thing. They question God and His will. They get angry or depressed and they think that they are the only people going through this. They feel alone and abandoned because their family don't know what to say. Honestly what do you say to someone that has cancer? I'm sorry? That sucks? Wish I could make it better? At least it isn't worse? We heard it all. We could answer them, you're sorry, why, did you make this happen? If not then don't be sorry. It sucks, yep, it does but we live with it. Wish you could make it better, not really because life has changed for us and that's okay. Then there is my favorite, at least it's not worse, really, why not just say, I'm glad you aren't dead yet.

Some people get so uptight about talking about having a spouse with Leukemia or Cancer but I keep it real. Does it suck, oh yeah. When you are established with a great doctor and insurance and medicine and then you either decide to move or you are forced to move or change doctors, insurance, etc. Do you sit down and cry? No, because you have to help find new places with great doctors or insurance and you have to make sure that the medicine and care continues. You don't have time for woe is me, because your family is counting on you.

One of the hardest times was about a year after he was diagnosed. He went to work and was told that they would not be able to keep him employed anymore because of his absences. The company that promised that they would work with him if he came back to work sooner than the doctor wanted was now telling him because he came out of remission and had to miss some work that he would be fired. Great the only one working while I was in college and homeschooling the boys was now out of a job. Also if he fought them on it they would fight his unemployment and his insurance. If not he would get his unemployment and insurance. Well that was pretty major to him so we couldn't afford to fight it.

After he lost his job, he went back in to remission in about a month. However, because the company called his firing a "mutual agreement" he couldn't find a job. No one wanted to hire someone who had leukemia and he had to disclose it because they would ask about the mutual agreement and he would tell them. At that point the interview is over. This went on for five years. He could not find steady work and because of my lack of experience and allergy to onions, I could not find work either. I couldn't work in restaurants or things like that because even smelling an onion makes my throat swell shut.

I thank God every day for my parents because without them we would be living on the street with no hope. They bought a double wide and put on their property and allowed us to live there rent free. They helped us with bills and gave us odd jobs to do to help. My parents have helped us more than I will ever be able to repay them. Because not only was there financial help they we there for us physically and emotionally.

Now I'm not saying that no one else helped us because I have an amazing mother-in-law who has been there every step of the way helping in any way she can. It's like when Doug was in the hospital the first time, she kept the boys so that I could be there with Doug and for Doug. I didn't have to stress about the kids because I knew they were taken care of. Even now she is there for us whenever we need her and has even traveled to South Carolina from Ohio just to help out. I don't know what I would do without her.

We have been blessed to have a very helpful and understanding family. They have given us the support and care that we have needed over the years.

We are also blessed to be able to work for a company that we believe in and believes in us. In the summer of 2014 we moved from Ohio to South Carolina for Doug to begin working for the Bluegreen Corporation, and it has been amazing. We live about a mile from the ocean and get to go to work for a great company every day. After the kids were in school and settled from the move, I started working for Bluegreen also and I love it. I get to go to work with my husband and best friend every day and we get to spend our drive talking and just being together. We learn so much more about each other because we have an hour a day just to talk and sometimes even vent about a bad day at work. It allows us that time that most people would spend once everyone is home to get things talked out and lets us devote our evenings and days off to our children and being a family.

When I tell people that I work with my husband, they say I'm crazy. I tell them that working together doesn't work for every couple but it works for us. He truly is my best friend and I don't know what I would do without him.